The Healthy Living Breakthrough

The Law of Nutrition And How To Change Your Life In Unexpected Ways

ROSSIE C PATTISON

CONTENTS

INTRODUCTION..i

CHAPTER 1 1

   EATING FOR HEALTH 1

CHAPTER 2 6

   PROTEIN FOODS...6

CHAPTER 3 9

   CARBOHYDRATES AND FATS 9

CHAPTER 4 12

   CARBOHYDRATES...12

CHAPTER 5 17

   NITROGEN TRICHLORIDE 17

CHAPTER 6 21

   FATS 21

CHAPTER 7 23

   WATER 23

CHAPTER 8 26

   VITAMINS...26

CHAPTER 9 30

   MINERALS 30

CHAPTER 10 36

   Calcium 36

CHAPTER 11 38

   PHOSPHORUS 38

CHAPTER 12 44

CHAPTER 13 47

   IMMUNE BOOSTING FOODS 47

CHAPTER 14 50

INTRODUCTION

With a great deal of heart disease being a direct consequence of a poor diet, a healthy life style is very significant in keeping a healthy heart. The most common type of heart condition is associated to high blood pressure. High blood pressure occurs when the blood circulation in your arteries are excessively powerful, creating little cracks. When they're repaired it prospects to the artery walls thickening and consequently results in problems with blood flow as well as a risk of clotting and blockages. Once the blood flow has reduced there is less of a supply to your vital organs, which creates dead tissues.

Research suggests that there is a strong link between nutrition and mental health, with a good diet having a positive impact. An innutritious diet is said to have a damaging effect on mental health with issues such as Alzheimer's, Attention Deficit Hyperactivity Disorder, Schizophrenia and depression – and their prevention, management and development.

There have been various studies carried out that suggest eating healthily can have a positive impact on mental health. By sticking to a balanced diet - with the right amount of essential fats, complex carbohydrates, vitamins, minerals and water – you can be assured that your mind and wellbeing will remain as healthy as possible.

Tryptophan, an amino acid, is said to improve your mood. It naturally occurs in protein and therefore, you should aim to have a source of protein with each meal. Foods that are high in protein include meat, eggs, milk, fish, nuts, cheese, beans and even some meat substitutes.

As well as eating healthily to maintain a healthy mind, mental exercises are also beneficial and there are many different ways to do this. Ideally, you should try and exercise your brain daily whether that is through doing crosswords, playing scrabble or even choosing not to use a calculator.

There are also various games that are specifically designed to exercise the brain. A recent research shows that there is a powerful connection between mental health and nutrition. A healthy diet can have a great impact on mental health with dilemmas like Alzheimer's, Attention Deficit Hyperactivity Disorder, Schizophrenia and depression - and their prevention, management and development.

There were various studies carried out that imply eating healthily can possess a positive impact on mental health. By sticking to a balanced diet - with the correct amount of essential fats, complex carbohydrates, vitamins, minerals as well as water - you can be assured your mind and wellbeing will remain healthy.

Tryptophan, an amino acid, is said to boost your mood. It naturally appears in protein and therefore, you should aim to have a source of protein with each meal. Foods that are high in protein contain eggs, meat, milk, fish, nuts, cheese, beans and even some meat substitutes.

Mental exercises are also essential and, as well as eating healthily to maintain a healthy mind there are various ways to do this. Ideally, you should try and exercise your brain daily.

Phytochemicals

Phytochemicals is a chemical compound that is found naturally in plants. It can be found in fruit and vegetables (broccoli, berries, apricots, onions, cabbage and so on), beans, whole grain cereals/ grains and even wine. Phytochemicals have different benefits depending on the type of food that they are found in, from acting as an antioxidant to preventing carcinogens from developing.

Antioxidants

Antioxidants are a substance that prevents oxidative damage.

They defend the body against free radicals – the result of a natural body process – that can damage healthy cells, changing the structure of   DNA resulting in tumorous growths. Antioxidants can be found in: Vitamin C which is in green peppers, oranges, strawberries (raw), red peppers (raw), papaya and broccoli.

Pro vitamin A can be found in cabbage, green spinach, carrots, collards, squash and sweet potatoes. Vitamin E which is in sunflower oil/ seeds, hazelnuts, almonds, peanuts and wheat bread. Omega-3 fatty acids Omega-3 fatty acids can be found in foods such as: kidney beans, flaxseed oil , soybeans and seafood – cold-water fish in particular.

CHAPTER 1

EATING FOR HEALTH

Like the man who defined love as "not beating your wife," nutrition is as much a matter of what not to do as what is proper. Nutrition is the science of keeping the body adequately fueled with the correct foods. Although eating should also entail the idea of pleasure, the chief importance of food is to keep the body cells healthy.

A cell cannot distinguish whether the protein it receives came from filet mignon or from beef stew; neither can the cell appreciate the gastronomic artistry of a four-layer cake piled high with frosting. In fact, if the cell could speak our language, it would probably shout, "For your health's sake, stop choking me with all those sugars and starches and send me more protein I It's not carbohydrates that make me happy, its amino acids!"

Because our cells were created in the knowledge of the "do's and don'ts" of good nutrition, it is about time some basis of understanding is reached between the mind that selects and prepares the food and the cell for whom the food is intended. Most of us would have nothing but the most genuine compassion for a young

4

infant before whom an ignorant mother would place a meal of ham, fried potatoes and strong coffee. Yet the things we do to our cells nutritionally make this gross ignorance look humane by comparison!

Proper nutrition is not as dreary a prospect as I once heard it defined by one teen-ager to another. "Nutrition," said the all-knowing adolescent, "means giving up everything you like sodas and hot dogs and stuff and poking down spinach and carrots."

On the contrary, nutrition can be a fascinating study. And certainly it should be one of prime interest to everyone, since it is so personal. I cannot eat for you; that is something we must do for ourselves.

Although we may have to depend upon other people to grow our food and to cook it, getting that food to the body cells its ultimate goal is something no one else can do for us.

That is why it behooves everyone to have at least an elementary knowledge of what constitutes good nutrition. Eating is far more than grabbing a bite to quiet a growling stomach. Like everything else, nutrition has its common sense side.

The best way to simplify a complex subject is to introduce it to you through its chief characters. Briefly, these are proteins (amino acids), carbohydrates (sugars and starches) and fats which, in turn, reduce to vitamins and minerals.

Water, too, is an important element of nutrition, although you may be accustomed to thinking of it as merely something to appease thirst, or to fill a bathtub!

Protein (Amino Acids)

Protein is a must in every person's diet, regardless of age. This being a nutritional axiom, it would seem that each of us would instinctively select enough of the protein foods that keep our human machine running in good condition.

But evidently we humans, with all our brains, are no smarter nutritionally than the laboratory rats in a recent experiment who were allowed to choose their own diet from various items set before them. Some of the rats ate wisely and were healthy, but their brothers and sisters failed to select the essential proteins and starved themselves into disease.

Dr. Scott of the University of Pittsburgh who conducted this test concluded from the results that if an intelligent animal like the rat would fail to select the right kind of food, it is even less likely that appetite alone is a safe guide for human beings.

The word protein means "holding first place"! And first place in the diet is exactly where protein foods belong. Amino acids (protein), not bread, are the staff of life.

Our bodies are made up of different kinds of tissues muscle tissue, nerve tissue, epithelial (surface) tissues, bone tissue and blood tissue, to name but a few of the more familiar tissues.

Each kind of the numerous tissues is composed of special types of cells muscle cells, nerve cells, skin cells, bone cells, blood cells. And each one of these various types of tissue cells is constructed of a material called protoplasm. Protoplasm is protein. Thus, our bodies are actually made of protein.

Did anyone ever succeed in trying to make steel with mud, or in attempting to repair an iron girder with putty? Of course not. In like manner, it takes protein to make protein, and protein to repair protein.

Perhaps I should say that it takes amino acids to make and repair body protein, since the different types of food proteins we eat are made up of different combinations of amino acids. And it is these amino acids, reconstructed into human proteins that build and repair the different kinds of protoplasm (protein) in our body tissues.

Therefore, good nutrition primarily means plenty of amino acids with which to build new cells and to mend ailing ones.

Each cell in our bodies contains at least eight different kinds of human protein. Some biologist has estimated that there are about 1, 600 different kinds of protein in the human body.

This means that the body cells require some 1,600 different combinations and groupings of the 23 amino acids, at least 10 of which must be contained in every diet based on good nutrition. Incidentally, I wish that the chemists had been foresighted enough to christen these vital body substances with a name more appealing to the public than "amino acids." I would have called them something like "cell builders" or "pep proteins."

We know that plants, too, contain protein. But plants can build up their proteins from the nitrogen in the soil and in the air; while man, like the other animals, must eat a form of plant or flesh protein, split it up into amino acids, and then rearrange these amino acids to form the 1600 different proteins which his body requires.

There are ten amino acids known to be absolutely essential to human health, that is, they must be contained in the daily diet, otherwise the work of the other thirteen amino acids cannot be completed.

Some of the other thirteen amino acids miscalled "non-essential" may come from the diet, while others may be produced within the body, since thrifty Dame Nature made it possible for our bodies to manufacture some of our own supplies of the thirteen "non-essential" amino acids, provided the ten amino acids were supplied in our daily food.

Yet, if even one of the ten essential amino acids is missing from our diet, the entire work of the other nine is disrupted. These are the "essential ten": arginine, valine, histidine, lysine, methionine, tryptophan, phenylalanine, leucine, isoleucine and threonine.

Among the remaining 13 amino acids now recognized and isolated is glutamic acid, the food element we have met in an earlier chapter as the substance that helps keep the liver healthy and nourishes the brain tissues, thereby raising the intelligence level.

CHAPTER 2

PROTEIN FOODS

The principal protein foods are lean meats (including glandular meats such as liver, heart, kidneys, brains and sweetbreads), fowl, fish, milk, cheese, eggs, beans and peas, whole grain cereals and nuts. Of these, meats, fowl, fish, cheese and eggs are classified as high-protein foods. To avoid a serious protein deficiency, at least half of the protein included in the daily diet must be obtained from these high-protein foods. Every twenty-four hours, a healthy person must have 4 to 6 ounces of protein rich food as an absolute minimum in order to avoid the serious consequences of protein-deficiency.

The demand for protein in the sick, ailing and convalescent body is, of course, greatly increased over this minimum figure. This absolute daily minimum of protein, if obtained from the low-protein foods such as grains, beans, peas and nuts, would not be sufficient to protect against a protein deficiency, since these low-protein foods do not contain all 10 of the essential amino acids.

Unfortunately, it often happens that some defect in the digestive tract such as low acidity of the gastric juices, or inadequate secretion of certain enzymes will hinder the splitting up of food protein into amino acids.

Many persons past middle age suffer from a serious protein deficiency, not because they do not eat enough protein foods, but wholly because their digestion is not efficient enough to break down the food proteins into amino acids, the only form in which the body cells can make use of protein. Hence these persons develop hypoproteinemia, meaning body lack of protein.

Drinking sweet milk with meals, or taking soda bicarbonate or other "alkalizers" after meals is one sure way to keep the stomach from doing a good, acid digestive job on the proteins eaten.

Nutritional science has hailed the production of concentrated amino acids with much enthusiasm because amino acids in this form are pre-digested protein, that is, protein already broken down into the only form in which the body can use food protein to build up its own types of body protein for the various tissue cells.

Especially did concentrated amino acids earn their medals in the days immediately following World War II. The problem of feeding Europe's millions of starving, emaciated peoples was not simply one of sending over meat and grain.

These people had reached such an advanced stage of malnutrition and protein deficiency that their stomachs were unable to handle solid protein foods; in other words, their digestive processes were so weak because of long disuse that protein food was passed from the body without being properly broken down and assimilated.

These wretched war victims had been so long on a starvation diet that their bodies were no longer able to take meat and cheese and bread and convert them into health-giving food for the tissue cells.

To restore these victims of malnutrition to the health and vitality which years of protein-deficient diets had stolen from them, pre-digested protein, in the form of amino acid concentrates, were rushed overseas.

Nutritional therapy took note of what could be done for victims of malnutrition by administering amino acids, and as a result many older persons with poor digestion, as well as those with ulcers of the digestive tract and those on restricted diets, have been benefited greatly by this valuable supplement to the diet.

Geriatrics, that branch of medicine devoted to the health of older persons, has found in amino acids one of its most effective weapons in fighting disease and debility among men and women of advanced years.

The sad part about a protein deficiency is that it can be concealed for a long time by overeating of starches and sugars. Because carbohydrates supply a readily convertible energy, the body keeps on for a time without a serious breakdown.

However, the day must inevitably arrive when the body begins to voice its protest against a scarcity of protein in the diet. And that protest takes the form of degenerating tissues and poorly functioning organs. In other words, the protest makes itself known as disease.

CHAPTER 3

CARBOHYDRATES AND FATS

*Why Carbohydrates and fats
are never a good substitute for protein*

Carbohydrates and fats do not contain a single amino acid. And amino acids are the only material from which the body cells can renew themselves. Any home owner knows what must eventually happen to a house that is allowed to go too long without repairs it decays and falls into ruins.

Comparing the body to a house, we might say that carbohydrates are one form of fuel that we put into the heating stove; but proteins alone are the materials the bricks, the paint, the plaster, the shingles which keep the house in good repair.

A body maintained on a high carbohydrate diet must eventually run down because a serious lack of the amino acids found only in protein foods has allowed the cells to go unrepaired and un-replaced for too long.

The main point to remember in this nutritional controversy of proteins vs. carbohydrates is this: Any person who eats enough protein need never worry about getting enough carbohydrates, since the body will convert protein into energy whenever needed.

Nutritional science has ample evidence to prove its statement that man can thrive on proteins alone, but cannot live on an exclusive diet of carbohydrates. The Eskimos who live within the frozen wastes of the Arctic Circle subsist entirely on a meat diet.

From the flesh of fish and animals these Arctic dwellers obtain the protein needed to keep their bodies healthy and vigorous in a land of incessant cold and hardship. This is possible, since the amino acids derived by digestion from food protein may be partially burned to provide body energy.

We know that the body has the power to convert amino acids into either body protein or energy sugars (carbohydrates). Therefore, protein is a complete food in itself.

Carbohydrates, on the other hand, are not so versatile, and can never replace the amino acids of protein in body metabolism. We know that a great number of war prisoners who died in Japanese prison camps perished because they starved to death on an all carbohydrate diet.

The amount of work expected of these miserable, undernourished prisoners was far too great for bodies that were rapidly deteriorating because of a total absence of protein in the diet protein that was urgently needed to repair their wasting tissues.

There is good evidence to prove that a return to an all-protein diet would lengthen man's life span far beyond the present three-score-and-ten: It was only when man turned from his pastoral life to that of grain farmer that he began losing his grip on longevity.

When our forebears raised their own flocks, thereby assuring themselves of a bounteous supply of meat and cheese, they lived far beyond the first hundred years without reaching the pitiful stage of senile degeneration which begins attacking modern man soon after his fortieth year.

But when man started drawing together with others of his kind into gregarious communities, forsaking his old nomadic life of following his sheep to fresh pastures, it was necessary for him to begin subsisting on food that could be obtained from the earth where he chose to remain.

It was then that man turned into grain-raiser and carbohydrate eater, and began writing his own death certificate at an age far earlier than that at which his ancestors had died.

And we, today, who do not even raise and eat our own grain, but who must depend upon farmers to till mineral-depleted soils and upon millers for devitalized white flour and upon vegetable and fruit raisers in far distant states for the carbohydrates around which we build our menus, die even sooner than the men of former centuries who subsisted on the fruits of their own lands.

If the human race is not to become progressively weaker, both physically and mentally, it must accept this nutritional truth: The only way to offset the artificiality of modern diets is to increase the protein intake to its maximum, and to reduce the carbohydrate consumption to an absolute minimum.

CHAPTER 4

CARBOHYDRATES

I find many people are confused as to exactly what carbohydrates are. After my lecture one evening, a woman assured me that she had eaten no carbohydrates at all since beginning to follow my health regimen. "We never use white flour or refined sugar anymore," she said, "only plenty of whole wheat flour and honey. We found carbohydrates were bad for our health."

"But any grain or any sweet is a carbohydrate," I corrected her.
"Oh, no," she insisted, "you told us only devitalized foods were carbohydrates."

It took quite a bit of further explaining to straighten out this woman's erroneous interpretation of carbohydrates. Carbohydrates in the human diet are divided into the sugars and the starches. The sugars consist of cane sugar (either white or brown, both of which are now devitalized completely of their natural molasses in the refining process to the point where they are worse than worthless as an item of the diet), syrups, molasses, and fruits either raw or cooked.

The starches include all flour (either white and unfit for human consumption, or whole grain and containing nature's own vitamins and minerals), flour products such as macaroni and noodles, breads, crackers, cereals, as well as starchy vegetables such as potatoes, beans, peas and parsnips.

All these various kinds of food carbohydrates are converted by the digestive juices of the mouth (saliva) and of the upper intestine into a body sugar called glucose. This glucose is absorbed through the intestinal walls and delivered directly to the liver via the portal vein.

A small portion of this glucose is converted by the liver into glycogen (the animal form of starch) which is stored in the liver to be reconverted into glucose body sugar as the system of glands and muscles may require this body sugar for energy.

Notice, please, that I said a "small portion" of this glucose is made into glycogen and stored in the liver. The remainder of the glucose derived from our high-carbohydrate diets passes directly into the bloodstream without being processed by the liver.

Why? Because the human liver was designed to handle only a small amount of carbohydrate, since man was primarily intended to be a carnivorous (meat-eating) animal. Therefore, the comparatively vast quantities of sugar and starch foods with which we insult our digestive system must necessarily prove far more than the liver is equipped to handle.

This is the reason why the body tissues are constantly receiving uncontrolled, imperfectly processed amounts of glucose directly from the digestive tract, instead of receiving correctly proportioned amounts of properly converted glycogen doled out to them by the liver as the need arises for this energy sugar.

Since we eat far more carbohydrates than the body needs for energy, what happens to the surplus amounts of half-processed glucose? They pile up as unwanted deposits of fat in the body in the abdomen, the hips, the limbs, around and in the heart, along the walls of the arteries and even in the liver itself.

More "fuel" pours into the bloodstream than the tissues can possibly burn for energy, and the surplus must be gotten out of the bloodstream in order to accommodate the steadily arriving fresh quantities of glucose.

Therefore this harmful surplus is stored as fat deposits anywhere that the body can possibly make room for it, regardless of whether or not such storage is harmful to the body's health.

Because I have mentioned several times that the glucose derived from carbohydrates is burned within the body to produce energy, please do not get the mistaken idea that only carbohydrates can furnish bodily energy.

To emphasize an important fact, let me repeat that when the amino acids derived from food protein are broken down, they leave what is called the carbohydrate moiety. This is a body sugar derived from food protein.

When this carbohydrate moiety that comes from food protein is burned within the tissues to produce energy, it gives a far hotter "flame" than either carbohydrate or fat. In fact, protein will burn with an energy degree comparable to 30 while the figure for carbohydrates is 6, and for fats it is only 4.

Thus we see that protein is a much better source of heat and energy for the body than either carbohydrates or fat. Most Americans are white-bread fiends. Bread eating, in itself, would not be so bad if it were not for the fact that the bread is made of flour that has been stripped of every vestige of natural food value through over-refining.

White flour is a devitalized food. Devitalized means exactly what it implies—"to deprive of life or vitality." Therefore, a devitalized food is one that has been robbed of the very elements which make it worthwhile as a wholesome, nourishing food fit for human consumption.

How many of the premature deaths among the 25 to 65 age group are caused by months and years of juggled diets meals which apparently include the "star! Of life," but which, in reality, provide nothing more than a poor grade of starch?

How many of the wasting diseases among very young children (the newspapers tell of these tragic cases almost every day) can be laid at the door of devitalized wheat, corn and sugar products to say nothing of synthetic colorings and flavorings in candies and soft drinks ?

A food may be "pure" and still be a fraud. The consuming public is subjected to such frauds in every pound of white flour, white refined sugar and devitalized corn meal. Millions of dollars are spent each year for magazine and radio advertising to extol the "wonderful food value" of white bread, pale-faced cookies and crackers, rubbery cakes and indigestible pies.

As I write these lines, the radio beside me has blared forth with this announcement: "Mothers, buy Miracle Bread for your children. More nourishment in each loaf than in a pound of steak, or two quarts of milk.

Contains ten vital food elements!" Where do these "ten vital food elements" come from? Certainly not from a flour which has been washed, scoured, screened, sifted, chemically bleached and milled until nothing is left but a constipation inducing starch.

Nature never created a white grain of wheat, or a white grain of rice, or a white grain of sugar! These improvements were left to the ingenuity of man.

How does white bread become white? It achieves this state of anemic perfection when the following elements are removed from the ground wheat grains: Three-fourths of the mineral salts and colloids, that is to say, three-fourths of the calcium, phosphorus, iron, potassium, chlorine, magnesium, fluorine, sulphur and manganese. Yet we are a nation of people admittedly mineral starved!

These minerals I have named are contained in the brown outer husk of the wheat grain, in the cells directly beneath this husk and in the germ of the wheat berry.

To produce "white flour," the mills sift and bolt out three-fourths of the minerals (plus an undetermined amount of the vitamins B-complex and E) leaving white starchy cells and the refined gluten of the inner grain.

What started this fad for white, refined foods? The profit motive, no less. Present flour milling methods were devised some fifty years ago for mechanical reasons because old stone-grinding methods were too slow, and also because white flour kept longer than whole grain flour.

Bugs and weevils cannot live for long in the devitalized product which is supposed to help sustain life in man and his offspring! It was certainly not dietary or hygienic reasons which dictated the present methods of milling flour, or grinding corn, or refining sugar.

Not only do the millers take out all the food value from the wheat grain, they add to white flour a harmful bleach called "agene" which is suspected of slowly poisoning its consumers.

Ninety percent of all white flour milled in the United States during the last 25 years has been bleached with a gene, chemically known as nitrogen trichloride.

CHAPTER 5

NITROGEN TRICHLORIDE

Nitrogen trichloride is a well-known nerve poison. One eminent physician has blamed this bleaching agent used in white flour as the cause of many nervous breakdowns, and of driving thousands of persons to alcoholism. One of Britain's foremost medical researchers, Sir Edward, was able to produce "running fits" or canine epilepsy in otherwise normal dogs within one to two weeks by feeding them a diet containing white flour bleached with nitrogen trichloride. Sometimes the fits became so severe that the animals died.

The experiment was carefully controlled at the British National Institute for Medical Research, so there was absolutely nothing else in the diet given these dogs that would account for this nerve disease except white flour.

Sir Edward declared that, during the present milling processes, ingredients definitely harmful to human health are added as preservative and bleaching agents.

During the bleaching process, a gas is generated and brought into intimate contact with the flour in a large agitator.

Although the gas is intended merely to bleach the flour, even the millers will agree that it "does affect" the gluten of the flour. What actually happens is that the chlorine of the gas reacts with parts of the gluten complex, leaving a poisonous chemical in the milled flour.

And, if the refining process should happen to result in darker flour than ordinary, more bleaching gas is used. This means a potentially more dangerous product than ever.

Following up the experiments conducted by Sir Edward, a group of United States Army doctors in Chicago duplicated the experiment using monkeys, since these simians are the most closely related to humans in their reactions to diet and disease factors.

The monkeys that were given the bleached white flour diet became sluggish, easily fatigued and inaccurate in judging distance when leaping to a new perch; and when they rested after being active for some time, they displayed marked tremors in the legs.

The results with the monkeys bear out Dr. Carlson's designation of nitrogen trichloride as a nerve poison. "This chemical," he said, "changes a good protein into a bad one and causes nervous instability. Very frequently such instability causes a person to become an alcohol addict."

In a recent issue of The Journal of the American Medical Association, the Army experimenters previously referred to declared that "agenized" (bleached) white flour should be investigated particularly as a possible cause of duodenal ulcers, the most prevalent type of ulcer in the digestive tract; for schizophrenia, a widespread form of mental illness; and for multiple sclerosis, a disease of the nervous system which leads inevitably to total disability, then death.

Agene converts gliadin, one of the proteins present in wheat flour, into a highly toxic substance. Even the small amounts of poisonous gliadin eaten each day in white flour products may, in time, result in slow poisoning of the entire body.

I can only wish that our Public Health Service would take as courageous a stand as did the British Ministry of Health when it warned that "flour should be the product of the milling of wheat without the addition of any foreign substance."

Perhaps all the hue and cry raised by these experiments will result in some sort of reform by the millers similar to that adopted by them when it became all too evident to the public that modern milling processes robbed the wheat of its food value.

After nutritionists had exposed the fraud of white flour for many years, the big milling companies finally came out with the "enriched" flour in a burst of radio and newspaper fanfare.

Public concern was lulled into a new lethargy by the highly touted claims that devitalized white flour had been "enriched" with some of the vitamins and minerals of which it had been robbed in a nutritionally criminal milling process.

Lepkovsky, reporting in the Annual Journal of Biochemistry, says that "if white flour is used, even if 'enriched,' it is difficult to see how deterioration of the national diet can be avoided."

In other words, so-called "enriched" flour is but a makeshift and an appeasement to public indignation at the commercialized ruination of good grain by stripping it of its food elements.

In a recent lecture, Dr. McCollum of Johns Hopkins said that the compulsory bread-enrichment program adopted by many states is not worth what it costs.

How much simpler and safer to give the public flour milled in accordance with the laws of nature which provides all food elements in proper balance when obtained from a natural source, instead of being distorted by commercially profitable refining processes!

CHAPTER 6

FATS

A certain amount of natural fat is necessary in a well-balanced diet. This fat should come from foods such as butter, vegetable oils (preferably olive, corn or peanut oils, since cottonseed oil is a high irritant to the digestive tract in some persons), cream, nuts, and cheese, as well as the fat contained in "lean" meat.

Fats in the diet have been given a bad name because the large amounts of carbohydrates in the diet take over the work of the fats in producing heat and energy, thereby allowing the fats to pile up in unwanted accumulations, principally in the arterial walls, contributing to hardening of the arteries.

After digestion, fats (now in a chemical state called neutral fat) are delivered directly into the circulation, by-passing the liver. Physiologists believe that the immediate destination of the fats is in the body tissue where they can be stored in controlled amounts against the time when needed to supply heat and energy for the body.

But the constant supply of sugars and starches that pour into our bodies do not make it necessary for the tissues to use up these fat deposits, so they remain in the body.

During periods of fasting or subsisting on a high-protein diet, the amount of fat in the blood plasma increases, since the absence of readily combustible carbohydrates forces the body to fall back upon its stores of fat in order to produce heat and energy.

This, in brief, is why we lose weight on a reducing diet the amount of fats and carbohydrates in the diet are so drastically reduced that the body must use up its stores of fat to supply itself with heat and energy.

My best advice to those who would live long, healthy lives, unencumbered by excess weight and free from the early menace of hardened arteries, is to burn up their fat, not allow it to deposit in the body.

This can only be done when the amount of natural fats in the diet is kept at normal, at the same time that the amount of carbohydrates is reduced to an absolute minimum.

CHAPTER 7

WATER

Despite the fact that water is scarcely, if ever, thought of as an element of good nutrition, it is a vital factor in good health. The human body can survive for many days without food, but it perishes within a very short time when deprived of water.

The many and varied chemical reactions described in this book as constantly taking place within our bodies all require water as the medium in which to complete themselves. For instance, the intestines cannot function normally without water, since this fluid is vitally necessary to the removal of waste products from the body.

That is why extra amounts of water should be drunk after a persistent attack of diarrhea or after taking a laxative to replace the water lost from the intestinal tract through the watery stools. Twice as much liquid is needed to complete digestion in the stomach and in the upper intestine as is contained in the entire bloodstream!

Over 75 percent of the body weight is made up of water in our tissues; more than half of this amount is found in the muscles, a fifth in the skin and one-fourteenth in the blood. The amount of water lost daily from the body via the intestines, the bladder, the sweat glands and in the breath, or abnormally from diarrhea and vomiting, must be replaced within a short time, otherwise the liquid balance of the body is disturbed, sometimes with serious consequences.

It is impossible to lay down an arbitrary amount of water needed by each person daily. Amounts will vary according to the person, the state of health and the season of the year. For instance, a person who perspires freely will need to drink more water in the summer when active than he will during the winter when leading a sedentary life.

This same person, moreover, will need far more liquid in the diet than a person who does not perspire easily and who sits out the summer in a cool place. Similarly, a person who urinates frequently and in large amounts will need to drink more water than a person whose urination is less.

Sometimes as much as 10 quarts of water are lost from the body by perspiration during extremely torrid weather, and two glassfuls are given off daily in all seasons through vaporization in the exhaled breath, with approximately five pints lost in normal urination.

From these figures can be realized the need to keep the body well-supplied throughout the day with water replacements. Generally speaking, the average person requires at least five pints of liquid daily. This may be taken as water, fruit or vegetable juices, milk, tea or coffee. Some liquid is also obtained from the food we eat.

While on the subject of water, let me caution that sometimes, in our zeal to follow a healthful regimen, we may drink water that is too pure. Distilled water should never be taken either by children or adults, except occasionally such as in the fasting program outlined for arthritics where mineral-free water is desired in the body to help absorb the excess calcium in the joints.

Water is a good source of minerals, and drinking water too free from minerals might lead to a serious mineral deficiency, unless these valuable food elements are supplied adequately in the diet or through mineral supplements.

CHAPTER 8

VITAMINS

The proteins, carbohydrates and fats we have been talking about contain mysterious food elements which we designate as vitamins, meaning necessary for life (vita). No one has ever seen a vitamin. But modern medical research has certainly seen hundreds of diseased results when vitamins are missing from the diet.

So much has been written and said about vitamins in the past few years that the public is becoming wearily indifferent to the subject, like the audience that tires of a song when it is sung and played over and over again.

It is unfortunate that the vitamin story has become so hackneyed, because it is one of the most important health stories ever told. The discovery of vitamins and the part they play in maintaining and restoring human health is one of the most important biochemical achievements of this age.

Thousands upon thousands of persons are alive and healthy today who otherwise would long ago have been laid in their graves were it not for the renewed lease on life given them by vitamin therapy.

The best way to present the vitamin story in order to avoid repetition and confusion is by showing them in relation to the work they do toward either preventing or relieving bodily disorders and diseases. This I shall do in the following chapter. Meanwhile, in brief, here are the vitamins now commonly recognized, and some of their principal food sources.

Vitamin A: Fish liver oil, liver, kidney, green and yellow vegetables, butter, cream and milk (unpasteurized), eggs, freshly ground yellow cornmeal.

Vitamin C: Citrus fruits (tree-ripened, preferably), melons, berries, pineapple, raw vegetables, raw fruits.

Vitamin D: Fish liver oil, liver, butter, eggs, raw milk. (This vitamin can be manufactured within the body by exposing the skin to sunlight. This is the only vitamin which may prove harmful in too large quantities. It is well to avoid all but very small doses of concentrated vitamin D, unless taken under the supervision of a competent physician.)

Vitamin B-complex: This group is made up of thiamin, riboflavin, biotin, niacin, pantothenic acid, choline, pyridoxine, folic acid, B-12, and several others either as yet not completely isolated or not tagged as to their specific function in the body.

All members of the vitamin B-complex group are found, to a more or less degree, in meats, both muscular and glandular, green vegetables, legumes, potatoes, whole grains, milk and eggs.

Vitamin E: Wheat germ, egg yolks, and the peeling and green outer leaves of vegetables.

Vitamin K: Green leaves of plants such as cabbage, spinach and alfalfa.

Vitamin P: Citrus fruits, especially lemons.

The amount of each vitamin present in natural foodstuffs is minute and immeasurable. Yet we know that when these minute quantities of natural vitamins either are destroyed by improper handling of the food or are withheld from the diet, very definite physical reactions make themselves known. Therefore, we know vitamins from what they do rather than from what they are or look like.

I take exception to the phrase "daily minimum requirement" which is used in connection with labels on vitamin products and in some articles written about vitamins.

Who is to say that the same "daily minimum requirement" of a certain vitamin will apply to all persons? Individual bodily needs make the "daily minimum requirement" a changing factor.

You may require far more of certain vitamins as a daily minimum than the arbitrary figure regularly publicized, and far less of other vitamins than the established minimum. The only reliable check on "daily minimum requirements" of all vitamins is your own sense of wellbeing.

When the food you eat satisfies you, is well digested, and leaves you properly nourished and glowing with a sense of health and wellbeing, then and only then can you be said to be obtaining a full quota of vitamins from natural food sources.

Unfortunately, however, far too many of us are deceived in the vitamin content of the food we eat. Ideally, the diet should supply the body with all necessary vitamins. Actually, it works out far differently.

Some foods do not contain the vitamins they should because of the way they are grown, picked and marketed; while other foods are robbed of their precious vitamin content because of poor storage in the kitchen or improper preparation.

I believe that the alarming increase in our so-called "civilized diseases" can be traced directly to the time when we stopped growing, processing and preparing our own food. There is little likelihood that pioneer families suffered any serious vitamin deficiencies.

They ate vegetables direct from their own gardens, either fresh or canned without benefit of vitamin-stealing preservatives; their bread was made of wheat and corn ground whole as needed; the milk they drank was not long from the cow's udder to the table so that the valuable vitamin A had not had a chance to be destroyed by heat and light as happens in bottled, pasteurized milk.

If we, like our pioneer forefathers, or our more fortunate neighbors who now live on farms or in small towns, could be assured of a supply of truly fresh foods, then I would say, "Forget about vitamins, and concentrate more on a properly balanced diet."

But the great majority of us must depend upon "store-bought" food for our tables, and we are forced to consider the all-important question of whether or not our diets contain adequate amounts of all vitamins to maintain maximum health and vitality.

For this reason alone, vitamin concentrates have been developed to make available an unfailing source of vitamins in definite quantities, thereby precluding the possibility of vitamin deficiencies in the diet.

Vitamins, in conjunction with their brothers in the family of food elements (minerals and amino acids), influence all the glands, thus affecting the production and activity of hormones in the body. So interrelated are vitamins, minerals, proteins and hormones that we cannot say one is more important than the other.

Like the instruments in a symphony orchestra, each food element has its place; when all food elements are present in the body in properly balanced quantities, harmony of health is maintained; when any one food element is missing, the discordances of disease are bound to arise.

CHAPTER 9

MINERALS

Lacking the dramatic publicity appeal of vitamins, minerals are the Cinderella of the food element family. Equally as important and equally as vital to good health, if not more so than the more "glamorous" vitamins, minerals nevertheless have remained quietly in the background, often being overlooked entirely by the person in search of good nutrition.

This is unfortunate indeed, since minerals just as vitamins and amino acids are vitally essential regulators and builders of the trillions of living cell units which make up the human body. Careful surveys of American diets reveal the discouraging fact that these diets do not contain enough minerals particularly calcium for optimum health.

Why do we need minerals? Because our bodies are literally a mineral quarry

In my reading the other day I came across this "Formula for a Human Being" as quoted by B. A. Howard in The Proper Study of Mankind: "Enough water to fill a 10-gallon barrel; enough fat for 7 bars of soap; carbon for 9,000 lead pencils; phosphorus for 2,200 match-heads; iron for one medium-sized nail; lime (calcium) enough to whitewash a chicken coop; and small quantities of sodium, magnesium, iodine, sulphur and other trace minerals.

Take these ingredients, combine them in the right proportions, in the right way, and the result, apparently, is a man." In the matter of blood, for instance, all that differentiates between human blood, plant sap and the "cold" blood of fish is a mineral; iron makes human blood red; magnesium makes "plant blood" green; and copper gives the in-between blood of the fish family.

Dr. Kahn says that if a human being were squeezed out like a lemon, no less than 11 gallons of sea water would be obtained, containing the same salts as dissolved in the ocean and in essentially the same proportions 80 percent sodium, 4 percent calcium, 4 percent potassium, and 2 percent magnesium, not to mention the numerous trace minerals found both in the human body fluids and in the ocean.

Minerals in the right proportions assure us of sound bones and muscles, strong teeth, steady nerves, a keen mind, firm skin and healthy organs. But few, if any of us look at our teeth and think, "Nice and strong.

That means plenty of calcium and phosphorus." Nor do we reason with ourselves when nerves get jumpy, "Jittery as a cat.
No doubt I've not enough calcium in my body." And rare indeed is the occasion when upon discovering that our skin, fingernails or hair are dry, brittle and aging, we say to ourselves, "Better do something about this. I need more sulphur."

I firmly believe that a basic knowledge of minerals and the part they play in maintaining body health is the first step toward a good understanding of nutrition as applied to everyday living.

Before I outline the minerals essential to good nutrition, I must make it plain that these minerals should be contained in the soils upon which our food crops are grown or grazed. But the soils of America, like the bodies of many Americans, are gradually being leached of their health-giving minerals.

Millions of acres of substandard soils are being cultivated to grow the grains, vegetables and meats which come to our tables in the guise of "mineral and vitamin-rich food," whereas actually these are underprivileged rations, since they have matured on soils that were too poor in minerals themselves to impart any of this mineral wealth to their crops!

It behooves every thinking American to read that startling book entitled Road to Survival written by William Vogt, the eminent scientist who does some plain talking about the rapid dissipation of the earth's topsoil through erosion and destruction of natural resources.

Vogt declares that by the removal of plants, forests and wildlife, and by over-cultivation, man has carried away important soil minerals and broken down the all-important mineral balance of the soil. After only fifty five years of cultivation, the virgin soils of Ohio, Illinois and Wisconsin (some of the richest farming land in the world) are estimated to have lost 36 percent of their natural phosphate.

More than 115,000,000 tons of topsoil, with all its vitally needed soil minerals, was carried off some 6,000,000 acres of rich Iowa fields by the July 1947 floods of the Missouri River. And many soils are so deficient in trace minerals such as boron, magnesium and copper that the plants grown on them have an extremely low nutritive value.

The crops grown on these soils, when they reach our tables, are but mere husks of the plant because the nourishing contents are not there. It is almost as though we bought a package of food at the grocery store only to find, upon returning home, that it was empty of its nutritive contents.

This matter of food for the flora and fauna of the earth is a never-ending cycle. We carnivorous or omnivorous animals eat other animals and plants which depend upon the soil for their nourishment; and the soil, in turn, depends upon certain plants, animals and bacteria for the minerals that make it fertile.

The basic materials of all soils are raw minerals. But poor management of the land, plus unwise plowing and planting methods that allow the minerals to be lost, is rapidly exhausting the productivity of our soil wealth.

Each year the same fields yield less and less; and each year the government finds it necessary to grant subsidies that compensate the farmer for his eroded, exhausted, mineral-leached soil.

But no subsidy can ever restore to the health of America the life giving minerals which ignorant, selfish and exploitative agricultural and timbering practices have stolen from our diets.

The only way to offset this serious mineral loss is for us to "subsidize" our own diets with mineral concentrates, to put back what rightfully should be in all food grown on well-tended, mineral rich soil.

There is such a wide variation in the mineral and vitamin content of the same types of foods grown on different soils in various sections of the country, even in different parts of the same field, that it is impossible to say that beets, for example, are a good source of iron.

Perhaps the beets in one end of the garden will contain a normal amount of iron, while the beets at the other end of the row in that same field will have iron content so low as to be almost negligible. Agriculturists recognize this fact.

In Illinois, for instance, some farmers refuse to buy corn from certain sections of their own state because those areas are notorious for their poorly managed or "worn-out" soils, meaning that crops grown on them are so low in food value as to be almost worthless.

Mineral loss from soils is not confined to certain areas of the country. Worn-out, mineral-poor soils are found all over the United States and from these deficient soils came the greater portion of the foodstuffs that reach the dinner tables of America.

Is it any wonder, then, that medical records show an alarmingly steady increase in degenerative diseases? I agree with Dr. Cavanaugh of Cornell University who said, "The fact is, there is only one major disease, and that is malnutrition.

All ailments and afflictions to which we may become heir are directly traceable to this major disease."

Why should malnutrition haunt us in a land where we enjoy the highest standard of living ever devised by man? We know approximately what constitutes good nutrition; we try to balance our diets; we adhere religiously to the dietary formula of meat, vegetables, fruits and whole grains. And yet we still are victims of malnutrition. Why? Because we have not learned, as yet, that no food is any more nourishing than the mineral content of the soil on which it was grown or grazed!

What can you do to insure yourself and your family against mineral deficiencies? I wish I could give you some quick, simple test to apply to the food that comes into your kitchen. Unfortunately, the food chemists have not yet discovered such a test.

The only way to safeguard against mineral deficiencies is to begin by suspecting that all food contains a more or less inadequate quantity of mineral value, unless that food is grown at home on soil which has been deliberately enriched by scientific methods.

From here, the next step is to provide the diet with concentrated organic minerals in amounts calculated to maintain body health. In that way only can we do something immediate to offset the laxity of the government in requiring that the soils of America be protected against the incessant loss of their invaluable minerals.

Luckily for us, these mineral elements necessary to the health of the human body are available in readily assimilable form at prices within the reach of nearly everyone.

I do not say that this is the ideal way to get our quota of mineral elements, but what other choice is left to us when the farmers and cattle raisers refuse to do anything to protect the soils on which they plant and graze the food we need to protect us against disease and premature old age?

About thirty different minerals have been recognized so far as making up the human body. More precious to us than gold or rubies are the "big two" of the organic mineral family calcium and phosphorus.

Without enough calcium, bones become weak and brittle, nerves are irritated, and muscles become flabby. The blood, spinal fluid, lymph glands and endocrine glands, as well as every tissue cell in the entire body, must have its full daily quota of calcium to remain healthy and to function normally.

CHAPTER 10

Calcium

Calcium may even be the key to a longer life. A recent experiment reported in the Journal of Nutrition reveals that laboratory animals which were given more calcium than needed for normal growth lived much longer than the animals receiving an "adequate" amount of calcium.

Moreover, it was noticed that the animals given the larger quantities of calcium reached a higher level of adult vitality and enjoyed a considerably extended "prime of life" as compared to the animals receiving only sufficient calcium to provide for normal growth.

Whether extra amounts of calcium will add years to human life, and prolong the health and vigor of the "prime of life," remains to be seen. Meanwhile, anyone who so desires may do his own experimenting, since calcium is a food element and not a harmful drug.

However, I must caution that any supplemental calcium added to the diet should be combined with sodium rather than being purchased in the form of pure calcium tablets, since the sodium assures that the calcium will be properly distributed in the body instead of being allowed to accumulate in the joints.

Calcium, invaluable food mineral that it is, can misbehave if sodium is not on hand to keep it in line. Those of you who depend on large amounts of milk to furnish your quota of calcium should also make sure to eat plenty of sodium foods such as celery and cucumbers, lettuce, apples, asparagus and squash provided, of course, that these fruits and vegetables were grown on soils not sodium-impoverished!

CHAPTER 11

PHOSPHORUS

Phosphorus "gets into the act" because it is the mineral colleague of calcium, and because a proper balance between these two minerals is essential before the bones, teeth, nerves and brain can benefit from the calcium in the diet.

This is another reason why it is foolish to rush out and buy a bottle of plain calcium tablets, thinking thereby to improve the health. Your money is wasted unless phosphorus, as well as sodium and other trace minerals, are also included in correct proportions. Phosphorus, either in foods or in concentrated form, is needed in ample quantities by all who do strenuous mental work.

A phosphorus deficiency may bring on loss of weight, general weakness, and mental sluggishness and reduced sexual powers.

Sodium

Sodium, in addition to acting as a "chaperone" for calcium, also helps prevent catarrh, as well as formation of stones within the gall bladder, kidneys and urinary bladder. A sodium deficiency may be marked by a death-like pallor, catarrh, deafness and a continual feeling of hunger.

Iron and its principal function in preventing or overcoming nutritional anemia have been discussed at length. However, iron is also needed for a normal complexion and to help maintain mental health.

People who are depressed and discouraged, who worry a lot, who suffer frequent headaches and whose memory is dull, usually need more iron in the diet.

Iodine

Iodine is the great gland regulator, since a serious deficiency of this mineral in organic form brings on goiter, leads to insanity through auto-intoxication and induces nervous breakdowns, as well as favoring obesity.

A high reserve of iodine in the body gives mental vitality and self-confidence, and prevents an abnormally rough, wrinkled skin and coarse lines.

Moreover, an iodine deficiency can contribute to stomach trouble and general debility. But please do not confuse mineral iodine with the liquid iodine sold in the corner drugstore.

The form of iodine needed by the human body is organic; it is found in seafood and in special diet supplements. No one should take medicinal iodine internally, unless prescribed by a physician.

Copper

Copper is a cohort of iron. It helps convert food iron into hemoglobin, the oxygen-carrying substance in the red blood cells that is needed in such abundance to avoid anemia.

A copper deficiency may be recognized by general bodily weakness and impaired respiration. Copper is also an integral part of certain digestive enzymes.

Potassium

Potassium is a versatile mineral, as well as a very important one. It helps maintain a normal heart beat and promotes the secretion of hormones. Because potassium regulates the normal contraction and relaxation of all muscles, it helps the movements of the intestines thereby preventing constipation or diarrhea.

In fact, that dread disease, acute diarrhea, which kills hundreds of new-born babies every year, has responded well to potassium which has reduced the deaths from this baby-killing disease to a very low figure.

Since diarrhea causes a high loss of potassium in body cells, restoring this mineral via concentrated form will offset a loss that can prove fatal if allowed to continue unrestored. Potassium also aids the kidneys to flush themselves of waste products, and it makes weak tissues more elastic.

Because of its influence on hormone secretions, a potassium reserve is especially important in the presence of female disorders.

Chlorine

Chlorine is the "laundryman" of the body. It helps remove poisons from the system by acting on the liver, that great filtering organ of the body. Chlorine is also necessary for production of enough hydrochloric acid in the stomach to assure proper digestion of proteins.

This mineral also aids in keeping joints and tendons supple, and takes part in distributing the hormones after their secretion by the endocrine glands.

Magnesium

Magnesium is called by biochemists the "cool, refreshing" mineral. It helps keep you calm and relaxed; it wards off undue discomfort in torrid weather by aiding you to stay cool. Magnesium is also necessary for all muscular activity; it activates certain enzymes for normal digestion.

This mineral also promotes normal bowel functioning, as well as the secretion and discharge of urine. A magnesium deficiency is often marked by abnormally wrinkled skin.

Manganese

Manganese (don't confuse this mineral with magnesium) is found only in trace amounts in the human body. But how vitally important those trace amounts are! Manganese nourishes the brain and nerves, aiding in co-ordination between nerve impulses and muscular action. In other words, manganese is one of the deciding factors between thought and action. It wards off neurasthenia and some forms of neuritis.

A serious lack of manganese is accompanied by dizziness, confused thinking, poor memory, unduly tender eyeballs, and poor muscular tone. Further, a manganese deficiency is suspected of being the decisive factor in lack of mother instinct. Laboratory animals deprived of manganese bore their young, and then promptly lost all interest in them.

But when manganese was restored to their diets, these females immediately started "mothering" the same offspring which they had abandoned completely only a few days previously.

Sulphur

Sulphur is called the "beauty" mineral because it helps keep the skin free of blemishes and makes the hair glossy. Sulphur also conditions the blood, making it difficult for disease germs to establish a stronghold in the bloodstream.

For this reason, sulphur is known as a systemic cleanser. Sulphur promotes secretion of bile and assists the liver in taking up other minerals. A sulphur deficiency is often accompanied by eczema and imperfectly developed hair and nails.

Silicon

Silicon is a great crusader in the body against tuberculosis and other serious diseases. It also helps prevent skin flabbiness and dull, expressionless eyes. Development of healthy hair, nails and teeth depends on silicon as well as on several other minerals.

Zinc

Zinc is concerned with normal growth processes, including hair, as well as with tissue respiration, that is, the intake of oxygen and the expelling of carbon dioxide.

Zinc is needed so the hormone insulin may be properly utilized, thereby preventing or aiding to control the disease known as diabetes. Indirectly, zinc is also involved in the body's use of carbohydrates. Greatest concentration of this mineral is found in the thyroid glands and in the sex organs.

Cobalt

Cobalt is another trace mineral whose presence is vitally needed for human health. Without cobalt, the normal blood formation cannot take place. When relatively large amounts of cobalt are included in the diet, the number of red blood corpuscles increases abundantly.

We first learned about the importance of this trace mineral when word came from Australia that sheep out to graze on certain lands began dying by the thousands of a peculiar blood disease.

After trying many remedies, it was finally discovered that the soil where these flocks were pastured was practically devoid of cobalt. When cobalt was given to the sheep in concentrated form, their blood disease cleared up at once. A similar experience was reported by a sheep raiser in Montana.

Boron has been revealed as the mineral with the specific task of controlling all cell growth. When cells are grown in soils seriously lacking in boron, they develop wild, uncontrolled cell growths that disrupt the life processes of the entire plant much as cancer does in the human body.

But when boron is restored to the soil, the plant growth from another crop becomes normal instead of developing wild, pulpy cells that crowd out and kill all efforts at normal development.

Translated into human nutrition, it is entirely possible that a serious deficiency of this trace mineral within the body may be partially responsible for tumors, cysts and other abnormal cell developments. Nickel, lithium, strontium and a number of others are "trace minerals" whose functions we have not as yet been able to tag exactly.

But we do know that trace minerals, however minute their quantity in our bodies, and have a special job to do. So important is that job that if the trace mineral is not on hand to perform, the body falls easy prey to some degenerative or diseased condition.

CHAPTER 12

Many of these trace minerals perform more than one specific task, and work in collaboration with vitamins, as well as with hormones.
The minerals, like the trace elements and the vitamins, work together in such harmonious teamwork that to disrupt the supply of one upsets the health rhythm of the entire body.

However, we do know that when vitamins are seriously lacking in the diet, the body is still able to make some use of its minerals. But when minerals are seriously deficient, vitamins are useless to the body.

Therefore, balanced nutrition means enough minerals so that full use can be made of the vitamins. This explains my greater emphasis on minerals. Dr. Sherman of Columbia University has said: "The importance of mineral salts in the tissues and fluids of the body is very great. Any considerable departure from normal is incompatible with life." Dr. Sherman further states that the average American diet does not supply enough calcium to meet all requirements of the body for this paramount mineral.

Dr. Rose, Professor of Nutrition at University of Illinois, says: "The chemical elements which make up the body sustenance must be nicely balanced or trouble ensues. The efficiency of each element is enhanced by proper amounts of the others."

Biochemistry has proved over and over again that our health can be no better than our mineral balance. That is why I urge you to pay more attention to minerals in your diet; otherwise you must continue suffering needlessly from mental upsets and physical ailments that have their only basis in mineral starvation of the body's cells.

Especially is a mineral-balanced diet important for persons after the age of forty. Elements such as phosphorus, calcium, sodium, iron, copper and magnesium exert a profound influence on the elasticity of the muscles and the strength of the bones, two bodily conditions which contribute much to the safety and happiness of old age.

Further, the mineral elements control passage of fluids from cell to cell; and they assist greatly in the digestion and assimilation of all food intakes, thereby relieving one of the most prevalent disorders of aging bodies. Minerals also aid proteins and vitamins to resist the onset of disease.

Calcium added to the diet of elderly persons may relieve the annoying itching that sometimes afflicts the aged skin. Because of its favorable influence on the contraction of the capillaries, adequate calcium is especially important for anyone with arteriosclerosis, coronary occlusion or thrombosis, or angina pectoris. Calcium is a tonic for the heart muscle.

In treating cases of chronic ulcerative colitis, calcium therapy gives unusually prompt results, acting to inhibit the bleeding and hyper-irritability of this very stubborn disease. Calcium has an important effect on bowel tissues that are subnormal because of disturbed nutritive conditions.

And, of course, broken bones heal much more readily when the calcium and phosphorus level in the blood is normal. But don't overlook the fact that sodium is also needed to control calcium in the body.

If you forget all else I have said in the preceding pages, remember this as the A-B-C of good nutrition: "The solid matter in my body is mainly proteins and minerals, and for that reason I must keep my body in good repair by providing it with enough of these vital materials."

CHAPTER 13

IMMUNE BOOSTING FOODS

Elderberry

Research has shown that an ascent remedy abstract from dark berries can block the flu viruses. However experts caution that supplementary research is required. Elderberry itself has the ability to fight inflammation and is also very rich in antioxidants.

Acai Berry

Acai berries also known as a "super food" are frequently found in in smoothie form or juice, dried and mixed with granola. This fruit is very high in antioxidants called anthocyanins. Antioxidants can also assist your body to fight disease and aging.

Oysters

Thanks a lot to the mineral zinc that's found in oysters. Oyster can significantly boost your immune system. Research has shown that male infertility is linked to low zinc levels.

Zinc seems to have several antiviral properties, granting researchers can't clarify why. Nevertheless, they do identify it is essential to a number of immune system responsibilities which includes healing the wounds.

☐

Watermelon

Energizing and Hydrating, ripe watermelon has unlimited glutathione, antioxidant. Recognized to help support the immune system to fight infection, glutathione can found in the red pulpy flesh near the rind.

☐

Cabbage

Cabbage is known to be a great source of immune strengthening glutamine. Start adding cabbages of any variety (Chinese, red, white) to stews and soups to add in further antioxidants and increase your meal's nutritional value. You can find cabbage very easily in the winter months and it is also very inexpensive.

☐

Almonds

Almonds has riboflavin and niacin, B vitamins, a few almonds can revamp your immune system and help you fight stress. A suggested 1/4 cup serving carries approximately 50% of the day-to-day suggested amount of vitamin E, which supports in boosting the immune system.

CHAPTER 14

A Life With Arthritis

If you can't avoid arthritis, at least learn some of the facts about your disease, and how to make life easier for yourself. An honest medical man will admit there is no sure cure for arthritis. The disease may be treated more successfully in the first year and yet even greatly advanced stages of arthritis have been known to become inactive with no treatment at all. Arthritis, the crippler, remains a medical puzzle.

More than seven million Americans are victims of arthritis in one of its several forms. Each year, 100 million working days are lost because of this disease.

Although we can measure the income and potential production lost because of arthritis, no statistics could possibly estimate the hours of mental and physical suffering that this disabling disease causes its victims.

Yet, because arthritis lacks the dramatic appeal of cancer or polio or heart disease, no nationwide campaigns are launched to raise funds for the research so urgently needed to relieve the suffering of arthritis patients in all age groups.

Arthritis is either the most over treated or under-treated disease that afflicts those sitting patiently in the doctor's waiting rooms. And yet every treatment is an experiment that may, or may not, bring relief.

The thought of a "cure" is too much to hope for, as yet. When the disease goes away, as it often does, it is seldom because of any one specific treatment. Arthritis is still as much a medical mystery as cancer.

We know what happens after the disease sets in, and we suspect some of the things that seem to bring it on or make it worse. But the exact cause, or causes, and the one specific cure are something still to dawn on the medical horizon.

However, from the experience of thousands of sufferers, we have learned some of the safe things that will bring relief. And we have also learned the potentially dangerous treatments to warn against.

The chief aim of any arthritis sufferer should be to learn how to live with his disease. The diabetic patient knows there is no cure for a degenerated pancreas, so he accepts the condition and learns to adapt his daily life to his incessant need for insulin and to his dietary limitations.

In like manner, the arthritic patient should first acquaint himself with the facts about all types of arthritis in general, and his own type in particular. He should learn the things suspected of bringing on this disease of the joints; he should observe his own case closely to determine what seems to help him most.

If it is a safe treatment, if it brings relief, he should continue using it despite the scoffing of those who "can endure your pain" bravely.

Most of all he should learn what to do, as well as what not to do, in the way of diet, exercise and mental attitude.

My sole purpose in writing this chapter is to attempt to provide a primer of common sense for the arthritic sufferer. It may help him to find the regimen that affords him the greatest relief.

Meanwhile, each patient can do his own research, so long as he remains within the limits of safety and common sense. And I will welcome reports as to their success from any who try the regimens I describe. Perhaps together we may hit upon the combination of things that will spell "permanent relief" for the more than seven million persons now wondering how to get rid of their arthritis. First, let's consider a cause for arthritis that has been given a lot of publicity lately. That cause is nothing more inflammatory than your own mind.

As long ago as the eighties, doctors spoke of "nerve causes" in connection with an attack of what was then miscalled "rheumatism," but which we now specify as arthritis. Time after time they noted the onset of arthritis as the result of an emotional shock.

They observed the pain and swelling grow worse in the presence of worry and fear. And they watched the acute symptoms subside as the emotions grew calmer. And because these medical men of that day knew little or nothing of bacteriology, they relied more on the "nerve" theory to account for arthritis.

Then came the era of germs and drugs, and the old "nerve" theory was dropped in favor of more tangible causes such as infected teeth, tonsils, appendix, sinuses, gall bladder or anything else that becomes infected in the human body.

A lot of teeth, tonsils and appendices were sacrificed in the hope of relieving arthritis. In some cases the disease showed an improvement after these drastic removals, but in equally as many cases no betterment was noted.

And now thousands of human parts later the "nerve" theory crops up again. Research in mental causes among 50 chronic arthritics at

Massachusetts General Hospital led to the observation that "poverty, grief and family worry seem to bear more than a chance relationship to rheumatoid arthritis."

Dr. Cecil of Cornell University Medical School states that "psychic traumas (emotional wounds), great and small, are of much more significance than focal infections" among arthritic patients.

Marital unhappiness, financial worries, grief, as well as long harbored resentments, loneliness and worry are suspected of supplying the spark that sets off the flame of arthritis in the joints.

There is a logical physical theory for the belief that sudden shock or continually overwrought emotions can bring on attacks of arthritis. We know that the sympathetic nervous system throughout the body responds to the slightest stimulus from the brain.

Therefore strong stimuli, such as those sent out by tense emotions, bring on disturbances of the blood vessels, causing them to go into spasm.

Medical men have long known that in atrophic arthritis^ the most disabling form of this disease, the circulation around the afflicted joints is greatly below normal because the capillaries (the feeder blood vessels) are so constricted that adequate blood nourishment cannot reach the inner tissues of the joint cells.

The tiny capillaries are found to be thin-drawn and almost bloodless. With their only source of nourishment dried up, the joint is deprived of the oxygen and nutritive elements needed to keep it functioning efficiently.

Try running an automobile motor without oil or water, and you will appreciate why a joint that is asked to "run" without proper fueling loses its smooth, satiny appearance, and why the bone "rusts," becomes brittle and breaks off in tiny flakes.

This theory that joints are damaged because an emotionally tense brain causes the nerves to close up the food "pipe lines" to the joint is a sensible one. It may be proved in some cases that infectious forces probably started the trouble in the first place.

However, allowing the capillaries to become constricted because of uncontrolled emotionalism is not going to give the blood a chance to send its germ-fighting equipment into the invaded area.

Harassing thoughts, whether they cause arthritis or merely aggravate it, are not going to make the disease any easier to live with.

A good mental housecleaning can probably avert more serious symptoms, or give a measure of relief from those already far advanced.

Arthritis selects women for its victims more often than men. Why, no one can say definitely. Yet the more tightly keyed nervous set-up in the female of the species would make this greater susceptibility among women quite logical, in view of the "nerve damage" theory.

Particularly has it been observed that the woman arthritis victim is usually slender and flat-chested with a prominent abdomen. Among the men who become arthritic, the long, lanky type seems to be most susceptible.

The terms arthritis and rheumatism have been so loosely applied that a great deal of confusion exists among the victims of these diseases as to whether they are "arthritic" or "rheumatic."

Arthritis is a general term applied to all inflammatory diseases of the joints, ranging from the slight form that may afflict an injured finger or ankle, and then clear up in a few days, to the type that renders its victims bedridden for years. There are about 100 different types of arthritis.

Rheumatism affects the nerves and muscles, and is also diagnosed in its different forms as neuritis, neuralgia, lumbago and sciatica.

Those 100 different types of arthritis fall into five classes:

• Traumatic arthritis, resulting from a blow, sprain or some other physical injury to the joint.

• Gouty arthritis, caused by a disturbance in body metabolism so that uric acid is retained in the tissues and blood, and then deposited as salt crystals in and about the joints. The joint most frequently affected is that of the large toe which becomes red, swollen and extremely painful.

• Infectious arthritis, caused by other diseases such as tuberculosis, syphilis or gonorrhea.

• Osteoarthritis (old-age arthritis), resulting in older persons from the wear and tear on the joints. As a rule, this type comes on gradually, and is rarely found before forty, although almost everyone who lives beyond the middle years will experience at least a touch of this type arthritis.

• Rheumatoid arthritis, the exact cause of which remains uncertain at this time, although we know that it is not primarily a disease of the joints, but rather a general disease of the system, of either organic or mental origin.

This last type, rheumatoid arthritis, is the crippling form of the disease. The joints not only become stiff, they gradually freeze into rigidity. Rheumatoid arthritis may come on suddenly with little or no previous warning symptoms.

Since it is a disease of the physical system, it may also involve the skin, muscles, heart, nerves, even the eyes, in addition to the joints. This characteristic involvement of other parts would point firmly at the cause in many instances as being due to a run-down physical system pushed so far beyond endurance by an emotionally tense mind that the entire system rebels.

The common symptoms are usually those of any general disease at the outset. Usually there is a low-grade fever accompanied by anemia, extreme fatigue and palpitation of the heart. At this early stage no changes are shown in the joints.

Later the joints will calcify; the tissue around them will become swollen and sore; in the later stages the joint narrows and cartilage is destroyed, leaving it rigid.

Obviously, early recognition of the disease before changes occur in the joints will have the best chance for permanent relief. Anyone who has reason to suspect that a tired feeling and sore joints are the results of something other than unusually strenuous physical activity should take immediate steps to build up the resistance of his entire body. You can't start too soon to ward off rheumatoid arthritis.

Other symptoms that may foretell the onset of any of the other types of arthritis are: numbness or tingling in the hands and feet; soreness in the middle joints of the hand; inability to hold articles, letting them drop easily; difficulty in holding a pen or pencil to write; sharp twinges in the hands or knees, lasting but a moment at first, then gradually becoming more acute.

These symptoms may, or may not, mean arthritis in any of its forms, but don't take a chance. Get the body into top physical shape as quickly as possible; keep it that way through following a sensible diet and a sane health regimen.

Arthritis often develops in women during or after the menopause, giving some confirmation to one theory that glandular disturbances, especially thyroid, favor the development of this disease.

Faulty posture seems to set the stage for the development of arthritis, especially in the spine and lower limbs. A pulled-in chest and a pushed-out stomach make a posture ideally suited for developing arthritis.

In this connection, you overweight persons would do well to get rid of those excess pounds, for you are almost certain candidates for arthritic knee joints.

When the body is overweight, especially when most of the excess fat is deposited in the middle section, the spine is forced to tip backward at the hips to support the abnormal load. This creates a chronic strain on the hips and knees, as well as on the spine itself.

Climate has a lot to do with encouraging the onset of arthritis in those whose bodies are already susceptible or who have paved the way for this disease by physical or mental excesses.

A climate that is cold and damp in winter, and hot and humid in summer, with sudden freakish, unseasonal changes from one extreme to the other; is certainly not the climate that brings comfort to already aching joints. Naturally, every arthritic sufferer cannot migrate to a warm, dry climate.

But they can take care to avoid getting chilled. Certainly air-conditioned buildings are no boon to the arthritic sufferer. Fatigue that has been allowed to reach the chronic stage has much to do with the onset of arthritis. Cases have been known to improve remarkably merely by putting the patient to bed for a good rest, and by supplementing the diet with large doses of thiamin, for starving nerve cells.

The only effective treatment for arthritis is to treat your entire system. I don't ask you to take my word for it; that is the substance of a statement issued by the American Rheumatism Association. Arthritis, like tuberculosis, demands a generalized treatment rather than concentrated attention on the affected part.

Any patient who permits treatment of his arthritis to be confined to a few injections and "some heat" is no wiser than the tuberculosis victim who would swallow a cough medicine, rub a stinging ointment on his chest, and let it go at that.

The only way to fight tuberculosis successfully is to build up the body so it can do its own fighting. That, precisely, is the only sane method of attack against arthritis.

Gentle massage and low-grade heat, however, are frequently soothing adjuncts to the general systemic treatment in most types of arthritis. I do not mean to minimize their part in helping relieve the pain of arthritic joints.

I do want to emphasize that anyone who is at all interested in trying to regain a fair degree of his former health must attack the disease from within, where its real cause lies.

Even the cases of arthritis induced by a tense mind can often be arrested when the brain is so fortified through proper nutrition, and dietary supplements designed to nourish starving nerve cells, that the mind can relax and create mental reserves to cushion it against shock or nagging worries.

The build-up diet for arthritics must contain plenty of such minerals as calcium, sodium (to keep the calcium from being deposited in the joints), phosphorus and iron. These are all minerals that contribute directly to the health of the joints, as well as to nerve and blood health.

Vitamins A, B-complex and C (which affects bone development and provides increased resistance to internal infection) in bountiful quantities are part of this diet to restore the entire system to normalcy.

Vitamin D is another food element that is of great help in treating arthritis, although there has been a tendency on the part of some physicians to over-prescribe this vitamin, the only one with which there is danger of an overdose.

Therefore, the safest way to obtain large enough doses of this very necessary vitamin is by exposing the skin to the sun at regular intervals, in carefully timed periods, so that the body can make and store its own vitamin D.

The arch villains in the eating and living habits of nearly all arthritis sufferers are the sweets, heavy starches, condiments, strong tea and coffee, alcohol and excessive tobacco.

Anyone suffering from any form of arthritis in any degree of severity should avoid the carbohydrates of rich desserts and candies as he would a chilling draft. This also holds good for all spicy foods, as well as strong coffee and tea, alcohol and tobacco.

Now for the actual treatment that may help your arthritis become inactive, and which certainly should make it easier for you to live with your aching joints.

Do not be misled into believing this to be some "miracle" method that will banish pain and suffering overnight, for the treatment is a long process, requiring the utmost patience and co-operation on the part of the sufferer.

If this sounds discouraging, remember that the mental and physical conditions which contributed to the development of the disease in the first place were probably years laying the groundwork for undermining the health of your joints. These long-time ravaging effects cannot be overcome in a matter of hours or days.

Much of the progress in this treatment depends upon the patient's age, weight, heart condition, previous living and eating habits. The latter are almost sure to be all wrong; for it is more likely than not that they helped bring on the arthritis in the first place.

Further, the amount of nerve energy, disposition and temperament of the patient, the environment in fact; almost everything in his life have a distinct bearing on the degree of recovery attained.

My sincere message to all arthritics is to "be of good cheer" rather than "arise and walk." A strong will to recover is more to be desired than any effort to rush the recovery. So called "overnight" results in the treatment of arthritis do not last.

Some years ago the premature announcement of prostigimine as a "cure" for arthritis brought no permanent relief to those upon whom it was used, and most certainly it gave rise to false hopes among the millions of sufferers who are praying for something quick to cure their tortured joints.

The sooner a patient in the advanced stages of arthritis realizes and accepts the fact that there does not as yet exist any "quick" or "permanent" cure for his disease, the more chance he has of an eventual recovery or a high degree of relief.

Too much stress cannot be laid on the value of obtaining as much rest as possible in treating arthritis. This is true especially in the several types of rheumatoid arthritis, because fatigue very likely was a prime factor in bringing on the disease in the first place.

Prolonged bed rest is usually advisable in treating the early stages of atrophic arthritis (the twisting, crippling form); while 8 to 10 hours in bed each night, plus an hour or two in the middle of the day is enough for victims of hypertrophic arthritis, since too much bed rest may aggravate the stiffness of the joints.

For this and many other reasons, it is imperative that the victim know exactly with which type of arthritis he is afflicted. Equally as important as the hours of bed rest are a good mattress and springs, for a sagging bed puts added strain on already weakened joints, as does faulty posture while walking, standing or sitting.

Moderate exercise taken with the consent of the physician familiar with your case is often beneficial. In the acute state of atrophic arthritis, however, any exercise should be limited strictly to very gentle movements of the afflicted joints, always stopping just short of the point where pain is felt.

In the more severe cases, even this gentle movement is forbidden. Simple exercises, where permissible, preserve the joint's ability to move, so that when the disease subsides the patient will not have lost the use of these joints.

Physical therapy, taken under the direction of a competent physician, has proved of great value in treating rheumatoid arthritis, as well as most of the other types of this disease.

Fresh air, too, is an important part of any treatment for arthritis. The more oxygen taken into the system, the better it is for the general health of the human body. And, too, fresh air and sunshine create a certain calming effect on a sick body that does not occur in any other surroundings.

An arthritic should at all times refrain from hurrying and worrying, which place unnecessary obstacles in the road to recovery. Weight plays a large part in treating many cases of arthritis. The overweight arthritic should reduce sanely; and the underweight patient should try to put on a few pounds.

Because simple anemia is an important factor when trying to avoid or to overcome arthritis, the diet should contain plenty of iron-rich foods such as apricots, raisins, prunes, broccoli, chard, egg yolks (provided there is no other systemic reason, such as gall bladder disorders or arteriosclerosis, for excluding them), dried lentils, mustard and turnip greens, watercress, lean beef and lamb, and liver.

All these foods will help bring the hemoglobin back up to normal, thus preparing the way for waging the campaign against arthritis from within. One of the most effective preparatory steps for starting the dietary treatment of arthritis is to fast completely for a day.

The logic behind this regimen is that a day of fast helps free the body of accumulated wastes, thus enabling the specific treatment to go to work unhampered by noxious substances backed up in the digestive and intestinal tracts, as well as in the liver and kidneys.

On the night before beginning the fast, take a small dose of a mild herbal laxative. This should be accompanied by plenty of water to expel all waste matter from the colon without causing panic in the peristaltic muscles due to the dehydration that usually accompanies laxative measures.

On the day of the fast, absolutely nothing should be taken into the system except pure distilled water. At least a glassful every hour should be taken.

Because it is distilled, and therefore not saturated with bacterial or inorganic mineral substances, this water will gather up and absorb certain impurities and unwanted matter in the body. Then at the end of the day, repeat the mild laxative dose.

In addition to continuing the cleansing of the kidneys and the intestinal tract, such a juice diet provides the ideal way to taper off the fast; the liquids will continue flushing the kidneys and the colon, while the fruit will furnish nourishment without overtaxing the semi-active digestive organs.

As a further benefit, the juice diet will help counteract hyperacidity, a prime necessity in treating arthritis. Then, for a week after the day of fast, the diet should be expanded gradually by eating citrus fruit oranges, tangerines, grapefruit, lemons, limes and apples, figs, pineapple, peaches, dates, berries, or any well-ripened fruit except bananas.

Continue drinking the distilled water. This diet regimen will change completely the tone of the intestinal flora (a desirable accomplishment in beginning any treatment for arthritis), and will also provide more solid nourishment in preparation for the balanced diet to be started at the end of the seven days.

Each night during the week of the fruit diet, a small dose of a mild herbal laxative may be found necessary, should the greatly curtailed amount of food intake cause some constipation.

At the end of this seven-day preparatory period, the diet may be adjusted as desired, but it must be adequate and well-balanced, as well as adapted to the caloric and systemic needs of the patient. One who is overweight should avoid fattening foods such as cream, butter or avocado pears.

The patient who is thin and undernourished should increase the amounts of good natural fats such as found in those foods mentioned above.

Generally speaking, the diet should consist of plenty of fresh fruit (except bananas) and vegetables (avoiding the gas-forming ones such as onions and members of the cabbage family, if the patient's activity is greatly curtailed), at least two glasses of fruit or tomato juice daily, seafood, fowl, lean beef and lamb, whole-grain cereals and unsalted butter.

Tea and coffee are strictly taboo, but a tea made of a mild herb such as fenugreek may be substituted as a beverage both at mealtime and in between meals.

I do not advocate the use of mint in any form, for it is irritating to the delicate membranes of the digestive tract. In many instances, because of the low vitamin and mineral content of the fruits and vegetables bought in the market, it may be necessary to supplement this diet with concentrates of vitamins A, B-complex and C, as well as the minerals calcium and sodium, phosphorus and iron.

If there is difficulty in chewing or digesting meat products, the protein level in the diet should be maintained by using amino acids in concentrated form.

You may have noticed that the diet recommended for arthritics are one in which all devitalized foods are "conspicuous by their absence." No white flour, no refined sugar, no white rice for the arthritic the same rule should apply to the diets of everyone, ailing or healthy.

There is a "cocktail" that has specific value in the diet for arthritis. It is a "cocktail" of either celery or cucumber juice, or, for a change, half of each may be combined.

Because of its high sodium content, this "cocktail should be taken liberally, since sodium acts as a solvent on the calcareous deposits forming in the afflicted joints. (Sodium, in fact, is the most important of all minerals in the treatment of arthritis.

It would be to the definite advantage of all arthritics to use a sodium concentrate especially is this recommended if enough of the "sodium-rich foods" are not included in the daily diet.)

Another good idea is to add the juice of a lime or lemon to a glass of distilled water and use this beverage for quenching the thirst.
If results are not immediately evident, do not become

discouraged. Along with good diet, adequate rest and a relaxed mind, you will also need large doses of patience and optimism. Yours is a stubborn disease, one which has taken months, even years, to develop.

While neither I, nor anyone else, can promise you a "cure," still I do want to emphasize that the general treatment program outlined above has accomplished encouraging results for hundreds of arthritics. So why not be faithful and cheerful and give this regimen a chance to do the same for you?

www.ingramcontent.com/pod-product-compliance
Lightning Source LLC
Chambersburg PA
CBHW070316290526
45791CB00003B/1137